tackling musculoskeletal problems

a guide for clinic and workplace

identifying obstacles using the psychosocial flags framework

Nicholas Kendall, Kim Burton, Chris Main, Paul Watson

Kindly sponsored by:

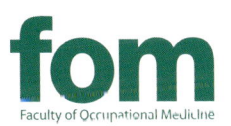

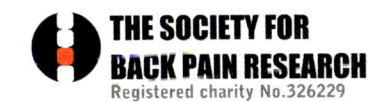

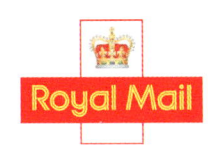

fom — Faculty of Occupational Medicine

THE SOCIETY FOR BACK PAIN RESEARCH
Registered charity No.326229

BackCare
The Charity for Healthier Backs

Royal Mail

hcml

Transport for London

London: TSO

TSO
information & publishing solutions

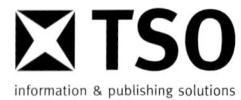

Published by TSO (The Stationery Office) and available from:

Online
www.tsoshop.co.uk/flags

Mail, Telephone, Fax & E-mail
TSO
PO Box 29, Norwich, NR3 1GN
Telephone orders/General enquiries: 0870 600 5522
Fax orders: 0870 600 5533
E-mail: customer.services@tso.co.uk
Textphone 0870 240 3701

TSO@Blackwell and other Accredited Agents

Customers can also order publications from:
TSO Ireland
16 Arthur Street, Belfast BT1 4GD
Tel 028 9023 8451 Fax 028 9023 5401

© Kendall & Burton 2009

Enquiries regarding copyright should be addressed to TSO,
St Crispins, Duke Street, Norwich NR3 1PD

The Publisher is not responsible for any statement made in this publication. Advice is offered by the authors for information only, and is not intended for use without independent substantiating investigation on the part of the potential users.

First published 2009

Second impression 2010

ISBN 978 0 11 703789 2

Printed in the United Kingdom for The Stationery Office

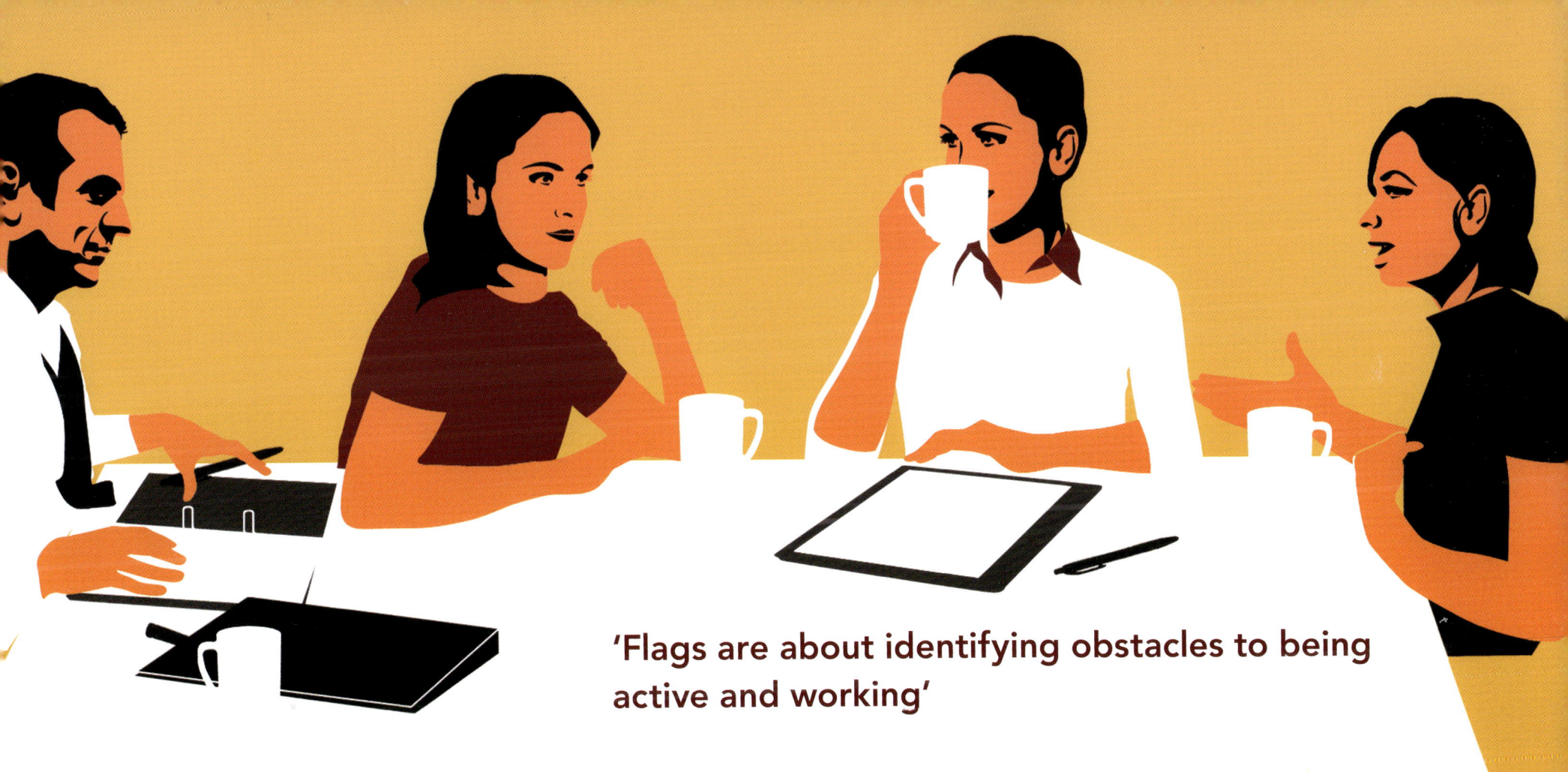

'Flags are about identifying obstacles to being active and working'

'The important thing is to figure out how these can be overcome or bypassed'

'Combining work-focused healthcare with an accommodating workplace is best: that means all players onside - consistency, coordination and collaboration'

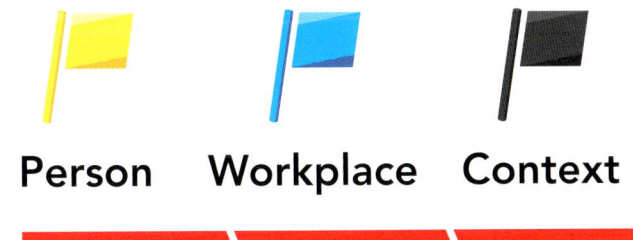

Person   Workplace   Context

identify flags › develop **plan** › take **action**

the flags think-tank

An international Flags Think-Tank was convened at Keele University, UK during September 2007. This two-day consensus meeting involved a multidisciplinary team of 21 experts in the psychosocial aspects of musculoskeletal disorders, and was followed by a one-day conference (Decade of the Flags) during which the deliberations of the think-tank exercise were presented to a critical audience. Following that feedback a number of academic papers, which form the evidence-base for this guide, were developed. The input to the guide from the Think-Tank participants is gratefully acknowledged as a material contribution.

participants

Mansel Aylward, UK
Kim Burton, UK
Peter Croft, UK
Mike Feuerstein, USA
Charles Greenough, UK
Elaine Hay, UK
Nick Kendall, UK/NZ
Clem Leech, Ireland
Steven Linton, Sweden
Patrick Loisel, Canada
Chris Main, UK (Chair)
Michael Nicholas, Australia
Ceri Philips, UK
Glenn Pransky, USA
Bill Shaw, USA,
Mick Sullivan, Canada
Danielle van der Windt, The Netherlands
Johan Vlaeyen, Belgium
Michael von Korff, USA
Gordon Waddell, UK
Paul Watson, UK

www.tsoshop.co.uk/flags

More information and resources for download are available here

contents

the flags think-tank	4
Participants	4
summary	6-7
workplace guidance	8-9
why and for whom?	10
the nature of musculoskeletal problems	11
the nature of 'flags'	12
Why Flags?	12
What are Flags?	13
Myths are obstacles	14
Uses for Flags	15
identifying flags	16
who identifies what and how?	18-19
important obstacles in depth	20
making a difference	25
action	26
Communication	27
Workplace accommodations	27
timing and stepped care	28-29
stepped care approach	30-31
advice for workers	32

Citation:

Kendall NAS, Burton AK, Main CJ, Watson PJ on behalf of the Flags Think-Tank. Tackling musculoskeletal problems: a guide for the clinic and workplace - identifying obstacles using the psychosocial flags framework. London, The Stationery Office, 2009

Illustrations and design detail by Rachel Oxley

tackling musculoskeletal problems
psychosocial flags for clinic *and* workplace

This guide is for everyone involved. Key players include: employers, clinicians, occupational health, and case managers

> The reason people don't return to being active and working is because they face obstacles
> Psychosocial obstacles can be more important than biomedical factors
> Flags are warning signals that psychosocial issues are acting as obstacles

This guide covers common musculoskeletal problems: not major injury or serious pathology

all players need to
- Identify Flags - they point to the obstacles
- Develop a plan to tackle obstacles - agree who does what and when
- Take action to help people get active and working - overcome the obstacles

to do list
- Remind the person that symptoms are common, and usually short-term. While some people need treatment, many settle with self-management
- Emphasise that activity is helpful, and prolonged rest isn't
- Don't tell the person work was the cause, it probably wasn't
- Remember most people can stay at work, perhaps with adjustment to tasks or schedule
- Take steps to achieve an early return to activity/work. It helps recovery, and usually does no harm
- Tell the person that long-term inactivity and time off work is detrimental to health and well-being

Key players can solve problems together to help the person get active and working by overcoming obstacles

Tackle musculoskeletal problems effectively by identifying flags and addressing obstacles - use a combination of work-focused healthcare and an accommodating workplace

> Helping people stay active and working is an imperative
> Address psychosocial issues promptly. Act sooner, rather than later
> Address both psychosocial and biomedical issues at the same time

identify flags
looking for obstacles should be a routine activity by all key players

why flags?
Flags point to obstacles in need of action

All players have a role in spotting flags related to the Person with the problem: their Workplace: and the wider Context of their lives

Help people by identifying obstacles to recovery and activity/work

when to look for flags
Start looking as soon as symptoms are reported or the person goes off work

Do it in steps - start simple, then delve deeper

everyone ask
- What do you think has caused your problem?
- What do you expect is going to happen?
- How are you coping with things?
- Is it getting you down?
- What are they doing at work to help?

everyone look for
- Lack of workplace contact during absence
- Inappropriate or unnecessary healthcare
- Contradictory approaches
- Delays in healthcare or workplace facilitation
- Lack of engagement or willingness to participate
- Progress undermined by relevant others

person

thoughts
- Catastrophising (focus on worst possible outcome, or interpretation that uncomfortable experiences are unbearable)
- Dysfunctional beliefs and expectations about pain, work and healthcare
- Negative expectation of recovery
- Preoccupation with health

feelings
- Worry, distress, low mood (may or may not be diagnosable anxiety or depression)
- Fear of movement
- Uncertainty (about what's happened, what's to be done, and what the future holds)

behaviours
- Extreme symptom report
- Passive coping strategies
- Serial ineffective therapy

workplace

employee
- Fear of re-injury
- High physical job demand
- Low expectation of resuming work
- Low job satisfaction
- Low social support or social dysfunction in workplace
- Perception of high job demand/'stress'

workplace
- Lack of job accommodations/modified work
- Lack of employer communication with employees

context
- Misunderstandings and disagreements between key players (e.g. employee and employer, or with healthcare)
- Financial and compensation problems
- Process delays (e.g. due to mistakes, waiting lists, or claim acceptance)
- Overreactions to sensationalist media reports
- Spouse or family member with negative expectations, fears or beliefs
- Social isolation, social dysfunction
- Unhelpful policies/procedures used by company

evelop plan
y players communicate

take action
stepped approach, just what's needed, when it's needed

ink obstacles!
Key players combine information to identify the important obstacles for this person, in this workplace, in this context
- Use written confidentiality waivers

evelop a plan
r the Person with the problem
- Tackle specific obstacles by taking specific actions
- Each Action has
  - agreed timeframe
  - a responsible player
- Emphasise ability
- All players
  - agree common goals
  - ensure accommodating workplace
- Copy of plan to all players and person
- Provision for revising plan

evising a plan
ck of progress, or lower level of activity d not returning to work indicate the need re-evaluate Flags and identify new or anging obstacles

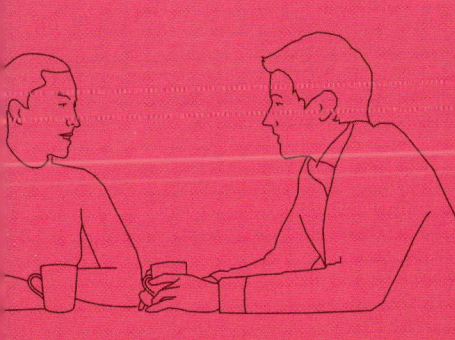

ctive and working
veryone has a role to play

	initial phase < 2 weeks	early phase ~ 2 to 12 weeks	persistent phase > 12 weeks
	Focus – symptomatic relief; maintain activity level	**Focus – early return to activity/work; everyone must have a work focus**	**Focus – optimal level of function; consider shifting goals**
	TIME FROM ONSET OR GOING OFF WORK		
healthcare	**always** • Provide advice to stay active • Reassure and give rational explanation • Advise person on symptom relief, and employer on work • Set realistic expectations • Dispel myths • Provide evidence-based diagnosis and treatment	**then add** • Select cases for psychosocial management • Use cognitive-behavioural principles • Provide a 'fit note', emphasise ability not disability • Reassure and explain typical pattern of discomfort • Liaise with employer • Suggest suitable modifications to enable RTW to begin • Cease ineffective therapy	**then add** • Maintain communication with workplace • Multidisciplinary programme that delivers cognitive-behavioural pain management and vocational rehabilitation • Avoid serial ineffective therapy • Emphasise self-efficacy
workplace	• Assign someone to keep in contact with employee • Address any organisational obstacles • Ask about any problems with work tasks or the way work is organised • If necessary, modify the work: temporarily reduce exposure to problematic elements • Encourage attendance at work meetings and social events • Educate and inform staff about effective return to work (RTW) approaches	• Assign responsibility to ensure RTW is discussed early, and implemented practically • Agree a RTW plan. Implement graded RTW plan • Obtain reliable (e.g. occupational health) advice if needed • Maintain regular contact • Encourage attendance at work meetings and social events • Use transitional work arrangements (modified work) to help early return to work • Continue liaising with other players to facilitate RTW • Review workers status with specialist occupational health provider • Reiterate workers worth to company	• Consider temporary re-deployment, or need for re-training
everyone	• Encourage activity & participation • Promote staying-at/returning-to work • Use workplace for rehabilitation • Dispel myths • Encourage self-management • Ensure timely healthcare access • Communicate with other players • Stay in touch with person • Facilitate communication	• Use problem-solving approach to tackle obstacles • Monitor progress objectively • Liaise with employer • Cease ineffective therapy • Consider 'light' multidisciplinary programme that delivers cognitive-behavioural pain management and vocational rehabilitation • Ensure timely start to RTW process • Emphasise ability, not disability	• Refine and adjust goals • Be alert for serial ineffective therapy • Seek input/help from other agencies

© Kendall & Burton 2009   Full guide: www.tsoshop.co.uk/flags

tackling muscle and joint pain
a quick guide for the workplace

You – the employer, line manager, or supervisor – have an important role to play: use this guide to help you help your colleagues

what

Most people get episodes of muscle and joint pain. The onset may be from physical activity but more often there's no obvious cause. Usually there is nothing to worry about: serious injury or damage is rare.

Recovery is expected, but the pain may recur. Back pain is a good example: activity is generally helpful – prolonged rest is not; most people get better and back to work quickly - but some hit problems.

Muscle and joint pain is very costly when people are off work for too long. The old approach of staying off work actually makes matters worse. Early return to work is usually beneficial.

But people need help to stay at or get back to work. And, it's not enough to rely on doctors and other clinicians - the workplace needs to be accommodating.

People often struggle to get back to work. It's usually not because of a more serious injury. It's because they face obstacles: things about the **person**, the **workplace**, or the **context**.

Manu's Story
HOW IT ALL GOES WRONG

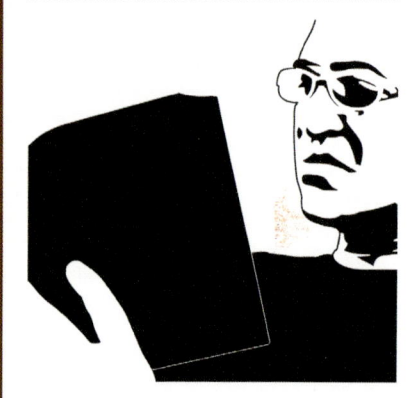

I got a back problem that made my work a bit difficult. The doc signed me off work, saying work probably caused the injury. The people at work didn't call, so I couldn't discuss getting back to work. The company have this rule that you have to be fully fit to go back - the pain kept coming and going so I was stuck. I got really worried and depressed. I don't get out much now and I've lost the job. To start with it wasn't too bad – all I needed was some help with the job for a while and I could have stayed in work.

identify obstacles

You can spot the obstacles by looking for flags – signals that things will get in the way. Mostly you'll be looking for workplace obstacles, but you need to work with the other players (doctors, health and safety reps, etc).

Identification is about looking for unhelpful behaviours and circumstances. Anything about the person, the workplace or the circumstances (including influential others) that stands in the way of early return to work is an obstacle.

myths are obstacles

These are all myths:

- Muscle and joint pain means something is seriously damaged
- Work/activity is the cause
- Time off work is needed as part of the treatment
- Cannot return to work until 100% pain free
- Contacting the absent worker is intrusive

What's the truth? Muscle and joint pain is very common, and often not caused by work, yet work may make the pain worse. Time off work is often not needed. Early return to work (with temporary modifications) is helpful. Funders, payers, & insurers support early return to work. Workers appreciate you staying in touch and having your support to get back to work.

identify flags ❯ **develop plan** ❯ **take action**

plan of action

goals: set a time for getting back to modified duties and to usual work.

can do? list can-do tasks and jobs (not just can't do)

obstacles: list what's getting in the way of getting back to work: job factors, personal factors, context factors – list who needs to tackle them

what and when? figure out the steps needed to overcome the obstacles, set a timeline: appoint someone to act as a support buddy/case manager.

how to act

Taking action is all about overcoming obstacles at work. It means providing an accommodating workplace, with helpful policies and coordinated actions. It's not rocket science!

- Contact the absent person within a day or two
- Tell them the workplace will be supportive
- Point out the return-to-work buddy who will be their case manager (perhaps the supervisor)
- Ask the person to come in to work to sort out the return plan
- Ask the doctor what the worker can do: Get their permission to talk with the doctor: use a confidentiality waiver (the worker gives explicit written permission for (selected) people to talk freely with the doctor/therapist)
- Assess the job, and offer modified work (if necessary) for a fixed period
- Allow graduated return to work plans, that offer gradual increase in hours and participation
- Monitor progress: revise the plan if any setbacks

modified work

Early return to work can be helped by simple modifications to the person's job. This is a temporary step simply to gradually ease them into usual work. Getting over the obstacles:

Alter the work to reduce physical demands: e.g. reduce reaching; provide seating; reduce weights; reduce pace of work/frequency; enable help from co-workers; vary tasks.

Alter the work organisation: e.g. reduced work hours/days; additional rest breaks; graded return to work; home working

Flexibility: e.g. daily planning sessions with a buddy; allow time to attend healthcare appointments; help with transport

---

Kamala's Role
The supervisor can make things happen

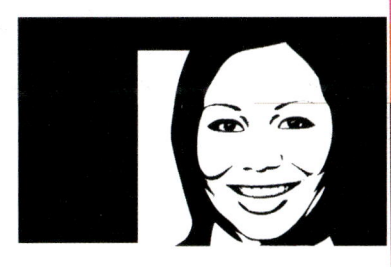

We're a small company with a simple protocol for managing pain and injury. It's my job to put it into action. Basically, I act as a case manager with support from professionals, to coordinate things. I get informed at day one of absence, and stay in contact. I liaise with the doc, but also send our people to a local clinic. They tell me what my colleague can do (we use a confidentiality waiver), which helps me figure out how best to help my colleague back to work. They point out the obstacles and what needs to be done to overcome them, as well as giving treatment. I devise the Plan with my colleague and we sort out any work modifications as a team. I also use information leaflets to help bust the myths. It works well!

© Kendall & Burton 2009   Full guide: www.tsoshop.co.uk/flags

why and for whom?

Most people experience musculoskeletal problems some time during their lifetime. They have considerable impact on individuals and their families. They are often a challenge to health professionals. The cost to industry, insurers and funders, the economy, and our societies is very high.

There is a paradox. Work loss due to musculoskeletal problems increased dramatically over the latter part of the 20th century – the very time when the physical demands of work were reducing and healthcare was improving! Most musculoskeletal problems are either a minor injury or occur spontaneously, so people should recover: fortunately they generally do and the experience is temporary. The trouble is that some people develop persistent pain and have substantial difficulty getting on with their lives.

Over the last decade we have learned a great deal more about how to tackle this predicament. We know at lot of what to do, but we're not always very good at doing it. This Guide explores the problems and solutions, and sets out the steps that need to be taken and, importantly, who needs to take them, and when. The principles for helping people recover return to activity are relevant for most people with common musculoskeletal problems: it does not address major injury or serious pathology. Therapeutic intervention for specific conditions should be provided: what is then important is facilitating participation – that is the focus of this guide.

Overarching Principles

- When people fail to recover and return to activity and work in a timely way it is mainly because **psychosocial** obstacles impede progress, not because there is more serious injury or disease

> *Psychosocial* refers to the interaction between an individual and their personal environment, and the influences on their behaviour

- Long-term inactivity and time off work are detrimental to health and well-being, so helping people to stay active or working should be an imperative
- The best way to tackle musculoskeletal problems is to identify obstacles and develop a plan to deal with them, sooner rather than later
- Overcoming obstacles needs action from the key **players**

Achieving **action** requires a number of simple steps

- Appreciation of the problem
- Awareness of the nature of obstacles
- Familiarity with the means of identifying obstacles – the Flags
- Development of a plan of action to tackle the obstacles
- Implementation of the action plan by all key players

Key Players

The two main environments where musculoskeletal problems can be tackled are healthcare and the workplace, so the key players are:

Healthcare - primary care practitioners, occupational health professionals, therapists, rehabilitation providers

Workplace - line managers/supervisors, senior management, human resources, health and safety advisors

The third concern is the person's context, the societal situation and system in which they function. This usually introduces additional players:

Context – spouse, family members, claims handlers, insurers, lawyers, case managers, employment advisors

> *Context:* Individuals exist in a variety of systems - the family system, the social system, the workplace or company, the culture, and the political system of the country in which the person lives. Collectively, these systems form the context for each person.

> *Players:* naturally the person with the problem is also a key player. However, this guide is focused on the clinic and workplace. It is assumed that everyone will encourage the person to accept responsibility to play their part

---

This Guide is for all the key players – it illustrates what to do, when to do it, and how to do it

The Guide explains the nature of psychosocial factors (*Flags*) and their role in development of pain-related restrictions in participation, productivity and work.

The *Flags* concept originated as a practical framework for understanding and evaluating psychosocial influences in musculoskeletal problems.

Flags are warning signals that psychosocial factors in or around the individual are acting as obstacles to full recovery and return to activities such as work.

The emphasis is on identifying *Flags*, then turning them into opportunities for action - combining appropriate treatment and management of psychosocial issues.

the nature of musculoskeletal problems

The term 'musculoskeletal problems' refers to the range of complaints and disorders commonly affecting the back, neck, upper limbs, and lower limbs. The plethora of diagnostic labels are characterised by pain, discomfort, and (all too often) disability.

The onset of symptoms may be sudden, and associated with activity, either trivial or strenuous. Onset can also be gradual with no identifiable triggering event. The causative mechanism is generally either unknown or unpredictable, so strategies aimed at preventing symptoms arising are destined to have limited overall impact.

Symptoms are often recurrent, but episodes tend to get better in a relatively short period of time – usually a few weeks at most. Most people return to work and usual activities with little or no help. For some, that expected recovery trajectory does not happen – symptoms persist and there is prolonged interference with activity and work – realigning the recovery trajectory is what this guide is about.

Symptoms may be accompanied by some measure of limitation in what a person can do, or feel able to do. Many aspects of life can be affected, including domestic and leisure activities, as well as work and interpersonal relationships. Persistent pain may lead to progressive withdrawal from activity and participation, accompanied by a sense of personal distress and uncertainty. Whilst some musculoskeletal conditions require specific medical intervention, the principle of facilitating participation by tackling psychosocial obstacles is relevant for all conditions.

Musculoskeletal problems are complex, both clinically and socially. Understanding and effectively tackling them necessitates a 'biopsychosocial' perspective. In recognition of this, the 'psychosocial Flags' initiative set out to develop a practical framework for assessing and tackling the wide range of factors that can act as obstacles to recovery and return to work. The core idea is the need to simultaneously address both biomedical and psychosocial issues.

'Work and activity are good for health and wellbeing'

- Musculoskeletal *symptoms* are a common experience: rarely does that denote disease or progressive pathology
- The symptoms are generally transitory, but are often experienced again
- Symptoms may be triggered by physical activities: minor soft tissue injuries are common, yet serious injuries and damage are rare
- Early recovery can be expected: specific treatment may be needed, although many episodes settle with self-management
- Activity is usually helpful; *prolonged* rest is not
- Seen overall, work is not the predominant cause, although the symptoms may be more pronounced at work
- Most people can stay at work (sometimes with temporary accommodations)
- Early return to activity and work can contribute to the recovery process: with appropriate facilitation it will do no harm
- Facilitating early return to work requires support from healthcare and accommodation at the workplace
- The best outcomes happen when key players share goals, beliefs and a commitment to coordinated action

Importance of maintaining participation, productive activity, and work

A higher level of participation in all types of usual activities is accompanied by higher quality of life, and lower level of distress.

Work is generally good for health and well-being. Long-term inactivity and time off work is detrimental. Helping people stay at work and return to work is, therefore, an important contribution to health.

For the majority of people, the most important consequence is not so much the pain, but the restricted participation.

Participation contributes substantially to the individual's quality of life. It also reduces the likelihood of long-term unemployment and the resulting negative health consequences.

the nature of 'flags'

Why Flags?

The essence of tackling musculoskeletal problems is not so much what has happened, but how to facilitate recovery and participation. Therefore, what is needed is a practical framework to underpin action.

Flags are a convenient way to group psychosocial obstacles to recovery and return to work. They represent a way of thinking about unfavourable outcomes in people with musculoskeletal problems and, at the same time, they indicate what needs to be done to improve those outcomes.

Flags have a dual role. They can help to select individuals likely to need additional help but, crucially, they also point to specific obstacles that need to be tackled.

There is consistent evidence that psychosocial variables influence the transition to persistent (chronic) pain, and the development of disability (limitations of activity and participation). Furthermore, psychosocial variables are stronger predictors of future pain and disability than medical/clinical factors.

Treatment using purely biomedical and biomechanical approaches has limited ability to resolve musculoskeletal problems. As the symptoms become persistent and often more extensive, with development of increasing negative effects and influences on the person, these treatments become less useful. Even before this stage, psychosocial factors can impede recovery. The evidence is clear that treatment directed simply at pain reduction does not necessarily result in improved participation and less disability.

Realisation of these various influences led to the 'biopsychosocial' approach to help explain and overcome the problem of unfavourable outcomes.

At the root of this approach is the important question: is it possible to redirect an individual's trajectory away from persistent pain and disability? In other words, can we identify people and situations where this problem is more likely, and can we do anything about it?

That is what the original Yellow Flags[1] were developed to achieve. The Flags concept has subsequently been expanded by the development of other types of Flags (Blue and Black), with increased focus on action to avoid unfavourable outcomes more than on their prediction. Care needs to be taken to avoid allowing Flags to be used as a reason to exclude the person from appropriate treatment or intervention.

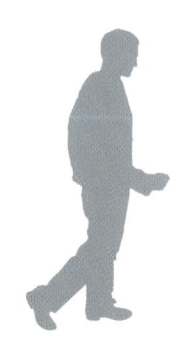

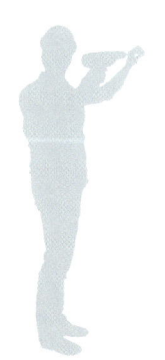

Flags *are*

Indicators that further attention needs to be paid to the presenting problem. This is usually in the form of more evaluation to ensure all potential obstacles are identified and understood.

An aid to bringing the biopsychosocial model into everyday practice. They offer an understanding of why some people with musculoskeletal problems don't recover as expected. They offer a method to identify and tackle obstacles to recovery or work.

Flags are *not*

Diagnostic: Avoid misinterpreting the term 'Flag' as synonymous with signs or symptoms. You cannot treat a Flag, it is a signal. You can determine if it indicates a specific obstacle to recovery, or to participation in productive activity. Obstacles can be addressed and can usually be overcome.

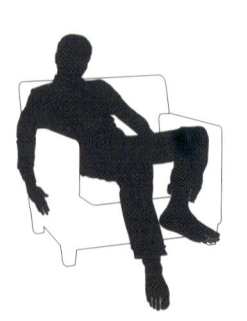

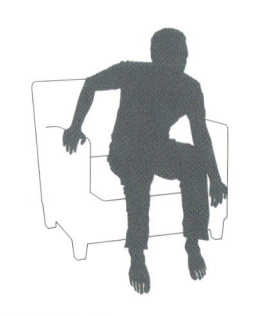

---

1 Kendall NAS, Linton SJ, Main CJ. Guide to assessing psychosocial yellow flags in acute low back pain: Risk factors for long-term disability and work loss. Accident Rehabilitation & Compensation Corporation of New Zealand and the National Health Committee, Wellington, New Zealand. 1997

What are Flags?

Flags are features of the person, their pain problem, and how they interact with the world around them. They can be identified by asking questions or making observations. Flags occur in three main domains and, for convenience, these are colour coded:[2]

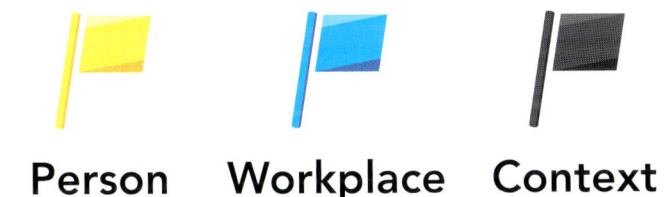

Person   **Workplace**   **Context**

The presence of Flags indicates an increased likelihood of an unfavourable course of recovery with respect to level of function and productive activity. They do not necessarily indicate the presence, or severity, of persisting pain.

Flags are not a diagnosis, and should not be used to label people - using Flags pejoratively defeats their whole purpose. Identifying Flags complements the diagnosis: their relevance is as contributors to the persistence of the problem.

A practical way to think of Flags is as 'obstacles'. Those that are modifiable can be overcome or got around. This perspective stresses 'ability' rather than 'disability', and shifts the emphasis to actions that facilitate recovery and return to participation. In this sense, obstacles can be transformed into opportunities. People usually need help to overcome or navigate round obstacles. This is where Flags come in – they point to the obstacles in need of action. Problem-solving approaches by the key players working together are often the most useful fruitful.

Describing the Flags

Detailed descriptions of the Flags are given later, but briefly:

Yellow Flags are about the person – they are largely psychosocial factors associated with unfavourable clinical outcomes and the transition to persistent pain and disability.

Blue Flags are about the workplace – they stem largely from perceptions about the relationship between work and health, and are associated with reduced ability to work and prolonged absence.

Black Flags are about the context in which the person functions, and include relevant people, systems and policies. These may operate at a societal level, or in the workplace. They are especially important since they may block the helpful actions of healthcare and the workplace. Contextual factors that cannot be changed need to be identified so that they can be navigated around. Black Flags indicate the potential need to involve relevant others and/or other professionals.

Multiple flags – psychosocial variables can have a cumulative effect - because the Flags interact, people often have multiple obstacles across domains – a Flag in one domain does not exclude one from another: rather it makes it more likely.

'What's important is appreciating how Flags contribute to creating an obstacle, and then working out how it can be overcome or bypassed'

---

2   In addition to the yellow, blue, and black flags, two other colours, red and orange, have been described. The concept of clinical 'red flags' is used across numerous medical fields including musculoskeletal disorders. They represent a simple set of observable parameters that alert clinicians to the possibility that the patient may have serious pathology or disease requiring investigation or urgent surgical referral. The 'orange' flags are the psychological equivalent of red flags. They serve to alert the clinician to possible serious psychological or psychiatric disorder that may render the patient unsuitable for a straightforward biopsychosocial approach. Acting as clinical decision aids, these flags are quite different from the yellow, blue, and black flags that form the basis for this guide.

myths are obstacles

Beliefs are central to our responses to an injury or a health problem, and influence what we do about it. Myths and legends abound, and are major obstacles to stay-at-work, return-to-work and vocational rehabilitation. Many of the Flags are related to these common myths. They are exceedingly pervasive, having negative effects on the behaviour of all the players, and the interactions between them. Myths need to be challenged and dispelled.

Myth	Reality	Why it matters?
Pain means serious damage and injury	- This is not always the case: pain can occur without injury. - Even when specific tissues are affected, activity and work are not precluded. - Temporary discomfort is often part of recovery.	- Believing hurt means harm results in focus on symptoms and activity-avoidance behaviours, which are obstacles for stay-at-work and return-to-work initiatives. - Worrying about 'damage' and 'injury' is an obstacle to active interventions that see work as a therapeutic intervention.
Work/activity is the cause: something's damaged	- Musculoskeletal pain is common across the whole population, regardless of type of work. - Work or activity can trigger symptoms, but most work is unlikely to cause substantial damage.	- Erroneously blaming work leads to an undue concentration on mechanical causation, which gets in the way of effective interventions. - Undue focus on mechanical workplace factors fosters the restrictive belief that ergonomic interventions are the only solution.
Work/activity will make matters worse	- The actual condition is usually not made worse by continuing work (assuming control of significant risks). - Work may become difficult or uncomfortable, but that doesn't mean it is doing harm.	- Work is generally good for health and wellbeing, so the belief that work is inherently dangerous is unhelpful, and poses a major obstacle to helping people get back to work or stay at work.
Medical treatment is necessary	- Most people, for most episodes of musculoskeletal problems, do not seek healthcare. - Reliance on healthcare alone is not enough to help with return to work.	- The beliefs of health professionals can fuel over-cautious behaviours, which are powerful obstacles to recovery and return to work. - Reliance on medical treatment alone negates the possibility of involving the workplace in helping people back to work.
Musculoskeletal problems must be rested	- Quite the contrary – activity leads to faster and more sustained recovery and return to work. - Temporary reduction of activity may be required, but long-term rest is detrimental.	- Using rest as a treatment is a major obstacle to modern management strategies that encourage and support return to activity/work. - Advising patients to take unnecessary rest can give the disadvantageous impression that the problem is serious.
Sick leave is needed as part of the treatment	- Often sick leave is not needed – staying at work is desirable, perhaps with some temporary modifications. - The use of 'fit notes' is preferable to sick notes: advise on what the person can do, not can't!	- Helping people stay at work can contribute to their recovery. - Injudicious use of medical certificates reinforces fears and uncertainty, and encourages reliance on rest, whilst fostering fears of activity.
Contacting an absent worker is intrusive	- Continued contact with the workplace is crucial to the return to work process. - If the approach is positive and un-pressured, workers are appreciative.	- Failure to make early contact with people who are off work leaves them isolated and unvalued, thus fostering distress or depression. - Lack of contact means these is no chance to make a return to work plan, and no chance to discuss transitional working arrangements.
No return to work/activity till 100% fit and pain free	- This is clearly unrealistic and unhelpful - many workers can and do return with ongoing symptoms, and they to come to no harm.	- Employers' policies that restrict work-return to those who are symptom free or fully fit for their usual work are counterproductive, and are a major obstacle.

uses for flags

The evidence indicates that identifying and targeting psychosocial factors has a positive effect, both on recovery and return to work.

Psychosocial factors can contribute during three stages of a musculoskeletal problem:

- before care-seeking
- at the point of seeking help
- as the problem evolves

The major value of Flags is as warning signals that the person is likely to face obstacles to recovery or return to activity/work. They indicate higher probability of persistent pain and difficulty with return to full independence and participation in usual activities (including work). Flags can be identified at any stage; delayed identification in the early stages increases the likelihood of more complex obstacles later on. That, in turn, makes subsequent attempts to tackle the issues much more difficult.

What is important is that people in the clinic and workplace consider all relevant factors. The Flags concept provides a framework to encourage and direct the search for obstacles. The consequence of not identifying Flags is that little or nothing is done to interrupt the individual's slide toward persisting problems, including the failure to stay at work or get back to work.

Identifying Flags and tackling obstacles is not the sole province of any particular group of professionals. A range of players is intrinsically involved in identifying and tackling them. This includes the person.

Having all players onside is crucial to obtaining good outcomes, and this depends on effective communication between them. The three Flag domains – yellow, blue, and black - are inherently linked and the effects interact. Managing one and ignoring others is less effective.

The Flags framework allows for the identification of obstacles and indicates the people who can take action to overcome them.

All the players must be onside: believing the same things; using a common language; having shared goals; coordinating their actions

---- without this, nothing happens.

Psychosocial factors

Psychosocial factors are more relevant to behavioural outcomes (including activity level, participation, productive activity, and work) than they are to symptoms (such as pain).

Sometimes the choice is between getting on and enjoying life or withdrawing from activity: either way, the amount of pain may well be the same.

When psychosocial factors are correctly identified and targeted, positive results can be expected.

Tackling psychosocial factors is not a replacement for appropriate treatment: is it a fundamentally important enhancement which can make the difference between effective and ineffective management. Tackling psychosocial factors needs to be intertwined with therapy.

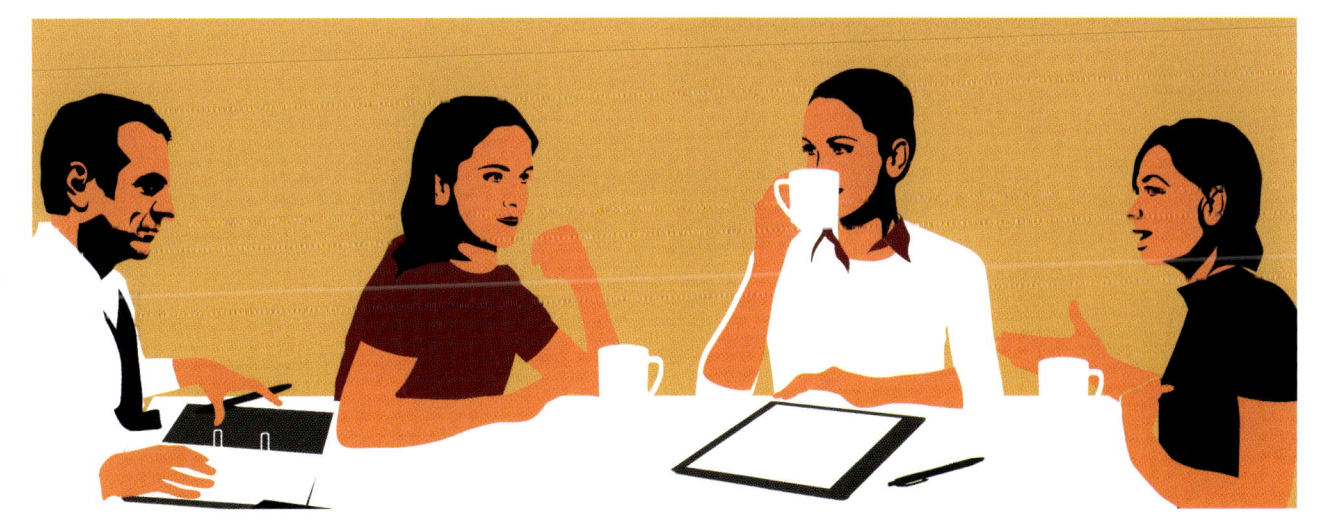

'All players onside – coordinating their actions to facilitate return to work'

identifying flags

how to evaluate the person, their circumstances, and the context

Looking for Flags should be a routine activity by all key players to guide the effective management of people experiencing musculoskeletal problems. This is essentially a matter of common sense and ought to be a straightforward process.

It can be useful to note the presence of psychosocial flags from the onset of the problem. However, more detailed evaluation is not usually necessary until a week or two has passed.

Psychosocial factors are part of everyone's daily life, and continuously influence us both positively and negatively. So it can be easy to see Flags waving everywhere! The critical issue is their relevance. The trick is to differentiate those that are important and in need of attention, from those that are irrelevant. It is a matter of seeking out those acting as obstacles to recovery and return to activity and work.

Identifying Flags depends on who you are and where you are – e.g. clinic, workplace, or community. Different players have different agendas, and the way they spot Flags will be different. For instance, supervisors have different skills and concerns from clinicians: the one is better placed to identify Blue Flags through observation of the workplace, whilst the other is better placed to evaluate Yellow Flags using structured interviewing. But, to successfully identify and evaluate all the relevant Flags needs a combination of perspectives.

Each key player has different opportunities to influence the person, and assist them with overcoming obstacles. But, because the various factors interact, it is essential that all the players are aware of the 'big picture' - Flags across the domains. Moreover, they need to be aware of, and make use of, contributions from the other players – this necessitates good communication!

Looking for Flags

Obstacles do not exist just in the person – they are also created by the surrounding context (the circumstances, and other people). Therefore various identification methods must be considered. There are three main techniques, and more than one may be needed:

Observation

- looking for unhelpful behaviours and circumstances (including looking beyond the person)

Asking open questions

- seeking less obvious Flags through direct interview (with the person, and relevant others)

Structured self-report questions

- identification of psychosocial factors using questionnaires (usually confined to the person)

These evaluation approaches may be thought of as a number of steps, with optimal evaluation always using more than one method. Invariably it will be necessary to talk to the person and make observations. Acquiring some of that information (e.g. descriptions of behaviours in other settings) from relevant others can be a very useful and objective addition.

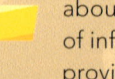

about the **person** - the major source of information is likely to be healthcare providers/clinicians.

about the **workplace** - the major source of information is likely to be the employer through the supervisor, human resources, or occupational health.

about the **context** - the major source of information is likely to be other relevant people such as family and spouse, employment advisors, case managers, social workers.

Ideally, information should be sought from all three important domains: the person themselves, the workplace, and the context in which the person functions.

As a reasonable rule-of-thumb, healthcare providers (e.g. physicians, therapists) can most easily obtain relevant information about the person (Yellow Flags). Employers (e.g. supervisors, human resources, or co-workers) can provide information about the workplace (Blue Flags). But, information can come from multiple sources – e.g. information about the person may come from employers and insight into workplace influences can come from clinicians.

In addition to personal and workplace factors, the person's context is important. These factors (Black Flags) may originate from the person's spouse or family, the social setting, the company, an institution or the social culture. Black Flags often represent organisation or system factors that the person finds difficult to navigate their way through or around without help or support. Everyone – including the person - should be on the lookout for Black Flags.

Importantly, the identification process is not a one-off exercise. Because the relevant psychosocial factors can change over time, re-evaluation of the Flags is likely to be necessary at different stages in the evolution of the person's problem. As different Flags emerge, they will point to different actions to overcome the changing obstacles.

Identifying Flags - Andy's story illustrates a host of obstacles related to the underlying perceptions and behaviours of the various players.

Andy's predicament

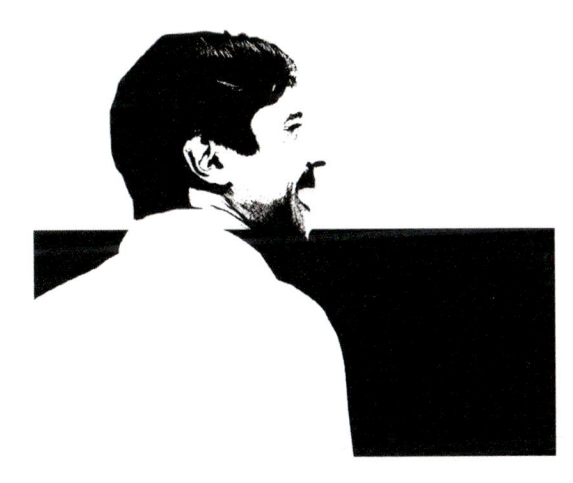

It all started when I woke up with severe neck pain. The doc gave me tablets and told me to rest and stay off work - but I didn't get any better. I was sent for x-rays, which showed degeneration. Then I had to wait around to get treatment. The therapist said it was my job that caused it, so I shouldn't go back till I was fully fit. By that stage I started to get really worried - and feeling down. The family won't let me do anything, so I don't get out much. The people at work haven't been in touch, so I don't know what's happening about me getting back. People are saying I should put in a claim. This whole saga has just taken over my life - all I wanted was a bit of help….

Using flags to select cases for targeted intervention

Preventing development of long-term disability and work loss depends on identifying Flags and obstacles, then taking appropriate action.

Identify flags > develop Plan > take Action

Identifying Flags is a way of selecting cases for intervention. In general, it is better to over-identify than to overlook people with the potential to slide into long-term problems. For example, facilitating return to work through workplace accommodation is preferable to extending sickness absence simply to 'play safe'.

Effect of overlooking cases – excessive suffering, risk of work loss and unemployment, high consumption of healthcare and potential for unnecessary invasive interventions.

Effect of over-identifying cases – unnecessary use of resources.

Conclusion - it is better to be over-inclusive so as to minimise the chances of missing a positive case, even at the risk of including more cases that turn out to be negative (false-positive). Selection measures need to have high sensitivity even if they have low specificity.

Note: interventions using cognitive-behavioural principles for musculoskeletal pain problems have no known adverse effects (so long as medicalisation and dependency are avoided).

who identifies what and how

Information about the…	Optimal evaluation method	Player most involved	Important obstacles to identify	Management implications
Person 🚩(yellow)	Stepped approach combining information from more than one method, usually in the following sequence: ○ Structured self-report ○ Open questions ○ Observation (Note: questionnaires can be used but they are not sufficient by themselves)	**Healthcare provider** Clinicians of all types Occupational health professionals	**Thoughts** Catastrophising (focus on worst possible outcome, or interpretation that uncomfortable experiences are unbearable) Unhelpful beliefs and expectations about pain, work and healthcare Negative expectation of recovery Preoccupation with health **Feelings** Worry, distress, low mood (may or may not be diagnosable anxiety or depression) Fear of movement Uncertainty (about what's happened, what's to be done, and what the future holds) **Behaviours** Extreme symptom report Passive coping strategies Serial ineffective therapy	Yellow Flags indicate a need for reassurance and positive advice. They also point to the potential need for approaches using cognitive-behavioural principles. ○ This means cognitive and behavioural principles are integrated into healthcare and workplace management. ○ It does not mean cognitive-behaviour therapy (CBT) per se is required. ○ This can be combined with other types of treatment and management.
Workplace 🚩(blue)	Stepped approach combining information from more than one method, usually in the following sequence: ○ Observation ○ Open questions ○ Structured self-report (Note: questionnaires can be used but they are not sufficient by themselves)	**Employer** Especially line managers or supervisors Human Resources, Personnel departments or occupational health professionals in larger companies	**Employee** Fear of re-injury Concern about physical job demands Low expectation of resuming work Low job satisfaction Low social support or social dysfunction in workplace Perception of stressful job demands **Workplace** Lack of job accommodations/modified work Lack of employer communication with employees	Blue Flags indicate potential need for enhanced workplace management, integrated with healthcare. ○ This means combining work-focused healthcare with an accommodating workplace ○ Communication with employee, graded return to work, transitional work arrangements (temporary) ○ Communication with healthcare to discuss return to work plan/person's needs
Context 🚩(black)	Combining information from both of the following methods: ○ Open questions ○ Observation	**Case Managers** **Employment Advisors** **Social Workers** **Relevant others:** spouse, family members, co-workers, etc	Misunderstandings and disagreements between key players (e.g. employee and employer, or with healthcare) Financial and compensation problems Process delays (e.g. due to mistakes, waiting lists, or claim acceptance) Overreactions to sensationalist media reports Spouse or family member with negative expectations, fears or beliefs Social isolation, social dysfunction Unhelpful policies/procedures used by company	Black Flags indicate potential need to involve significant others and/or other professionals. Influences within the person's social milieu (both private and professional) can sabotage progress. ○ This means care is needed to ensure a consistent approach by all players

Issues for everyone to consider	Communicate and share information	Develop a plan for action
The most important issue is for each Key Player to assess the overall situation, in addition to understanding the role of the other players: coordinated action is needed.	Ensure that all Flags and obstacles are identified through sharing relevant information (use a written confidentiality waiver). Ideally one person will collate information and coordinate communication. This rarely happens unless a specific person has been allocated – in the absence of a professional case manager, one of the players needs to take this role.	Evaluating Flags is about (1) early identification of issues that indicate increased probability of ongoing problems, (2) using that information to target appropriate intervention/support to overcome obstacles to recovery. This amounts to selecting individuals who have relevant Flags present. Each person with Flags needs an individualised Plan that outlines specific actions.
Everyone should be alert for • lack of engagement or willingness to participate • progress sabotaged by significant others • lack of workplace contact during absence • inappropriate or unnecessary healthcare • delays in healthcare or workplace facilitation • contradictory or counterproductive approaches	The importance of communication, especially between the workplace and healthcare cannot be overemphasised. Scenarios to avoid: ○ one player expecting another to take full responsibility for all aspects ○ contradictory approaches through ignorance of what other players are doing ○ delays while hoping another player will solve the problem Facilitate activity and return to work through: ○ conducting an evaluation of Flags and obstacles ○ devising a Plan for Action	Developing a Plan: ○ based on identification of specific Flags ○ directs intervention at overcoming the obstacles that are flagged up ○ outlines specific goals (measurable, achievable, with timeframes) ○ ensures all players share the same expectations ○ identifies who is responsible for each Action ○ describes an audit trail (so that all players can tell whether goals have been achieved, or how progress toward them has been made) ○ allows for revision or modification of goals when required Given the lack of adverse consequences it is better to provide interventions such as information, coping skills and problem-solving training, than not (within available resource constraints).

Interactions between Flags - Sam's story shows how systems obstacles can become person obstacles

SAM'S STORY

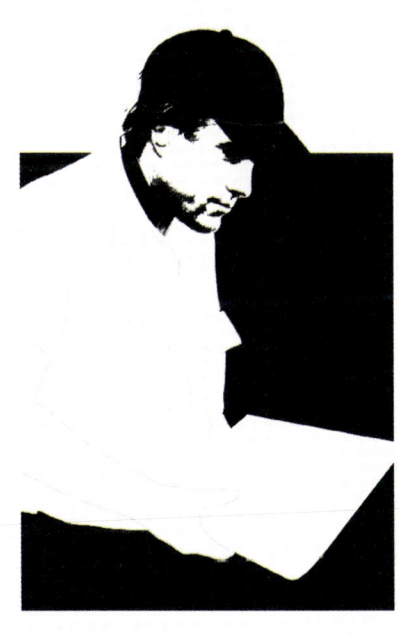

I hurt my knee when this guy just drove into my car. He apologised at the time, but then disputed the insurance claim. Naturally I was really angry. I mean, it was clearly his fault, and it was me that got injured not him. My solicitor said I should claim for the injury and all the inconvenience: that suited me – why should people like that get away with it! Obviously can't do a lot and have to keep seeing the doctor, but the solicitor says I'll get more compensation the more disabled I am. Clearly, going back to work simply isn't an option until this is all settled.

important obstacles in depth

The following Flags are frequently encountered and are powerful obstacles to recovery and return to work. The information amplifies that in the preceding table, structured to cover:

- definition
- explanation
- evaluation
- questions
- management

The list is not exhaustive, and it is expected that the Flags will be evaluated and tackled by personnel in the workplace and the clinic who are familiar with musculoskeletal pain problems. A crucial first step in all instances is provision of evidence-based information, including myth busting and practical advice, irrespective of specific Flags.

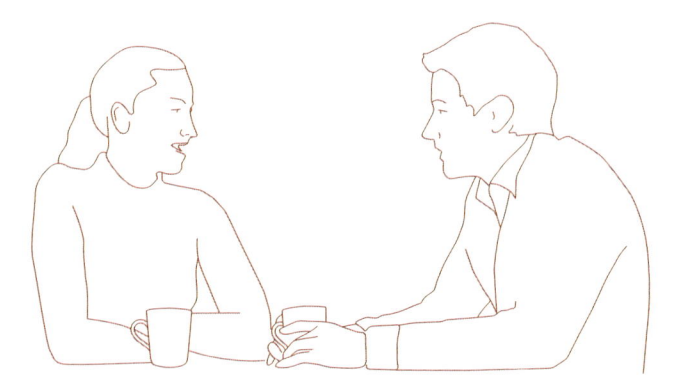

Catastrophising refers to a form of distorted thinking where the person focuses on the worst possible outcome, however unlikely, or interprets a situation as unbearable or impossible when it is really just uncomfortable.

Catastrophising can occur when a person feels pain, or expects to feel pain. The effect is to increase pain and suffering, to disrupt adaptive coping, to increase avoidance behaviour, and to allow unhelpful patterns such as a "boom and bust" activity cycle to develop.

Evaluation: Identify interpretations of symptoms, bodily sensations, or the person's situation that are out of proportion and that lead to a sense of unease and a lack of feeling in control.

Q1: When you are in pain do you think it is terrible and will never get better?
Q2: Does pain feel overwhelming to you?

Useful Management Strategies: Structured activity scheduling, and progressive goals; Cognitive therapy approaches such as positive self-statements or planned distractions, identifying and dealing with unhelpful thoughts; Thought-monitoring and cognitive-restructuring; Relaxation training.

Belief refers to the psychological state in which an individual holds a proposition or premise to be true.

Expectation refers to a belief centred on the future, about what is considered most likely to happen. (see also the section "Negative expectation of recovery and return to work")

We hold beliefs and expectations about most things in the world and this includes pain, activity, work, and healthcare. Beliefs lead to our emotions and drive much of our behaviour. Expectations shape our beliefs. When expectations are unrealistic (either unduly pessimistic or optimistic) this can lead to changes in our behaviour. Beliefs strongly influence our experience of pain, and when combined with expectations can significantly modify how we behave when we are in pain.

Evaluation: Identify unhelpful beliefs such as: that pain signals harm or damage; that pain signals the need to stop activity; that pain must be completely absent before activity is commenced; that pain is uncontrollable; or, that others are responsible for the person's recovery and rehabilitation. Identify unhelpful expectations such as: the prediction of increased pain with any activity; or, a sense that pain is unpredictable.

Q1: What do you understand is the cause of your pain?
Q2: What are you expecting will help you?

Useful Management Strategies: Cognitive therapy approach; Education and reassurance; Structured activity scheduling, and progressive goals.

Preoccupation with health refers to an excessive preoccupation or worry about having a serious injury or disease. It is anxiety about one's health.

Preoccupation with the fear of having, or the idea that one has, a serious injury or disease is usually based on a person misinterpreting symptoms or sensations. The effect can be treatment-seeking behaviour, and unwillingness to contemplate returning to activity and work.

Evaluation: Identify fear of injury or disease, despite negative findings and reassurance by clinicians. This might also be expressed as a lack of satisfaction with previous treatment, help and support from others.

Q1: Do you worry that you might have something wrong that hasn't been found?
Q2: How helpful have others been to you already?

Useful Management Strategies: Education and reassurance; Cognitive therapy approach; Structured activity scheduling; Graded resumption of activity and work.

Worry and Distress refer to feelings of unease, apprehension, suffering, or unhappiness. These are quite normal feelings that we all get from time to time. They may arise from unhelpful thoughts or expectations, as well as aversive situations. They may be recognised as irrational or excessive by the person experiencing them, but the person may feel s/he has trouble stopping or controlling them. If this is the case, they can create a risk that the person may do things to deal with them that end up being counterproductive.

Worry and distress are aversive states that may lead to maladaptive responses. They may occur in response to a specific event or stimulus, or be a person's general outlook on life. They may be the result of the behaviour of others, or because of beliefs and attitudes held by the individual. They can influence a person's expectations of the future (eg. by making predictions of what might happen – usually negative in nature). The effect can be to increase pain severity, to disrupt relationships and activities of everyday life, and to cause behaviours such as avoidance to develop. Behavioural excesses may occur if a sense of desperation emerges. Examples include taking too much medication, burning skin while trying to control pain with heat, or guarding a part of the body from movement.

Evaluation: Identify strong feelings of unease, apprehension, or worry, and what triggers these. They may be more significant when accompanied by a feeling of suffering and being unable to cope due to perception of little or no control over the experience of pain and its intensity. They may not meet criteria for a clinical disorder. Instead they may indicate the early stages of a disorder, be a sub-clinical problem, or be due to an underlying coping style (personality).

Q1: Have you been feeling worried or distressed?
Q2: What seems to trigger these feelings, if anything?

Useful Management Strategies: Cognitive-behavioural approach to address unhelpful thoughts; Stress management training; Relaxation training; Information and reassurance; Coping skills training, and practicing coping skills in a variety of real-world settings.

Depression refers to lowered mood that is often described as sadness or 'feeling down'; but, may be expressed in other ways such as helplessness, loss of interest, and frustration or agitation. The person does not always recognise the change in their mood, although it may be obvious to others.

Depression may occur in response to an event such as loss and grief, but can also occur without a specific trigger. It has both physical and psychological aspects, and can occur along with other diseases or injuries. The effect of depression can be to amplify the perception of pain and cause disturbance in important daily functions such as sleep, eating, and usual activity.

Evaluation: Identify strong feelings of sadness, loss, despair, guilt, apathy, and/or grief. These may not meet diagnostic criteria. Instead they may indicate the early stages of a disorder, be a sub-clinical problem, or be due to an underlying coping style (personality).

Q1: Have you been feeling low or down recently?
Q2: What do you think about your future?

Useful Management Strategies: Cognitive-behavioural approach (with/without medication); Computerised CBT; Structured activity scheduling.

Fear of movement or re-injury refers to the belief that moving specific body parts, or engaging in activities, will exacerbate pain and cause injury. The response is to avoid movement and activity. This can involve detrimental guarding specific parts of the body from all movement, and seriously impedes participation.

Fear of movement can become significant, akin to a phobia (described as 'kinesiophobia'). The effect on willingness and ability to participate can be significant, leading to substantial loss of quality of life.

Evaluation: Identify guarding of any part of the body, or avoidance of specific movements or activities. Also identify use of extended rest.

Q1: When pain increases does it indicate that you should stop what you are doing?
Q2: Are there any specific movements or activities that you avoid?

Useful Management Strategies: Merely advising or telling people to resume activity or work participation is insufficient when the person is fearful; identifying what the person is fearful of then providing an incentive to confront and overcome the fear is necessary. Effective treatment for fear of movement (kinesiophobia) can be obtained by desensitising the person to a hierarchy of their fears associated with movement and activity. Fear of re-injury may be general, or specific to the scenario associated with onset. Examples include fear of getting back in a motor vehicle following an accident, or climbing a ladder after a fall.

Uncertainty refers to doubts. This could be about what's happened, what's to be done, and what the future holds.

Uncertainty can arise from a variety of scenarios. For example, the person may have experienced conflicting diagnoses or explanations; they may have been exposed to diagnostic language leading to fear or catastrophising, such as a fear of 'ending up in a wheelchair'.

Evaluation: Identify concerns and lack of clarity held by the person.

Q1: Do you feel you have a clear understanding of your musculoskeletal pain problem?
Q2: Is any aspect of your problem especially worrying to you?

Useful Management Strategies: Education and reassurance; Cognitive therapy approach such as positive self-statements.

Extreme symptom report refers to the person rating severity at or above the top of the scale. An example is rating pain severity at "12 out of 10" on a 10-point scale. It is usually considered to be an expression of distress, and a method of communicating this. Sometimes it is a way for a person to make their invisible experience of pain more visible to others.

Extreme symptom report as a method of communicating distress indicates the person does not feel their problem has been taken seriously, by significant others. This might include spouses or family members, employers or managers, and healthcare providers. The effect of extreme symptom report can be to over-sensitise the person to whether others believe them about their experience of pain, and to the development of maladaptive behaviours. These usually need to be modified, using behavioural techniques.

Evaluation: Identify behaviours being used to express how distressed the person is feeling.

Q1: What is the worst your pain has been in the last week?
Q2: How do others respond to you when the pain is especially severe?

Useful Management Strategies: Education and reassurance; Distress management (see relevant section); Involve relevant other as rehabilitation 'collaborator'; reinforcement of 'well' behaviours.

Passive coping strategies refers to reliance on external sources of control over the pain; contrast with active coping strategies that are based on internal sources of control.

Coping refers to the cognitive, emotional and behavioural strategies people employ in their day-to-day attempt to manage their pain problem. Passive coping strategies include resting, hoping the pain will just go away, and catastrophising. Active coping strategies include exercise and productive activity, diverting attention, ignoring sensations, reinterpreting pain sensations, coping self-statements, and increased behavioural activities.

Evaluation: Identify passive coping, but ensure these are not due to compliance with treatment or instructions from others.

Q1: Do you still do things, despite the pain?
Q2: What do you do when you are having a really bad day?

Useful Management Strategies: Coping skills training; Cognitive-behavioural approach; Problem-solving skills.

Serial Ineffective Therapy refers to the delivery of sequences of treatments that yield little or no actual benefit to the person. These may occur because the person seeks them, or because the healthcare provider is over-enthusiastic in providing interventions.

Serial ineffective therapy results in negative consequences, adversely influencing both beliefs and behaviours. These in turn influence outcomes, such as failure to return to activity and work. Messages received by individuals receiving serial ineffective treatments: There is a problem that needs medical or physical treatment; Treatments will cure the problem; Symptom reduction is necessary first, before returning to activity; The healthcare provider is responsible, and patient merely has a passive role.

Evaluation: Identify history of either (a) excessive demand by person for treatments, despite lack of effect. Includes requests to see many healthcare professionals; (b) provision of multiple types of interventions and repeat treatments despite lack of effect; or (c), both of these. Be sure to check the effect on both the symptom severity and the effect on level of function and productive activity.

Q1: What treatments have you received, and how effective were they?
Q2: Have any treatments made a difference to what you can do?

Useful Management Strategies: Cease ineffective treatment.

High physical job demand refers to jobs with especially high or sustained biomechanical exposure: the 'problematic' level of exposure will be lower for symptomatic workers. Note that job demand may be subjectively perceived, or involve actual high loadings, or a mixture of both.

Evaluation: Identify job characteristics, and the individual's concerns about them: look for inflexible work schedules that do not allow appropriate breaks.

Q1: What types of tasks and activities does your job entail?
Q2: How is an average working day structured?

Useful Management Strategies: Transitional work arrangements such as work rescheduling, or part-time work with graduated increase; Seek alternative work only if return to same-job-same-employer is definitively impractical.

Negative expectation of recovery and return to work refers to the belief that the person is unlikely to get better and get back to work. This contributes to a sense of helplessness and undue pessimism. It is often associated with two types of mismanagement: (1) a focus on symptoms by asking people how they are feeling instead of asking what activity they have been doing; and, (2) a focus on what people 'can't do', rather than what they 'can do'.

Negative expectation leads to low self-efficacy so the person lacks a sense of mastery over their pain problem, and this often encourages passivity and a steady downward spiral toward low activity levels. Restoring a sense of optimism can be achieved through ensuring the person attains goals, progressively in steps small enough that success can be guaranteed.

Evaluation: Identify pessimism about recovery and return to work. This may be a belief that a certain period of time needs to elapse before the person feels better, or that some intervention (e.g. surgery) needs to happen before they can contemplate working again.

Q1: Do you think that your pain will improve?
Q2: Do you think that you will return to work?

Useful Management Strategies: Cognitive therapy approach; Emphasise ability (not disability); Structured activity scheduling; Graded resumption of activity and work.

Job satisfaction refers to how content an individual is with their job. Low job satisfaction or job dissatisfaction can reduce the likelihood the person will return to work when they experience a pain problem.

Many factors can contribute to job satisfaction and these may require careful questioning to clarify. They may include a range of personal factors (life goals, home situation, history); and workplace factors (interactions with co-workers, supervisors).

Evaluation: Identify job satisfaction with respect to factors such as work routine, management, salary, possibilities for promotion, and co-workers.

Q1: How satisfied are you with your job (taking into account the factors above)?
Q2: What aspects of your job are most dissatisfying?

Useful Management Strategies: In the first instance, discuss with employee, and try to find mutually acceptable changes to the work content, it's organisation, environment or culture; if all else fails, consider discussing a job change through job placement advice.

Low social support or social dysfunction in the workplace refers to the person's perception that they lack support from other people, at home or at work or both. Sometimes there is a degree of interpersonal conflict in the workplace.

The most common interpersonal difficulties encountered by people with musculoskeletal pain problems are (1) frustration or anger expressed toward them, perhaps as a consequence of their symptoms or inability to engage in activity or work; and (2) over-solicitousness, where a significant other is over-helpful in a well-intentioned way but ends up inadvertently encouraging activity avoidance and unhelpful beliefs.

Evaluation: Identify the perception of low level of support from the person's social network. The actual support may be adequate, but it is the perception that is important. Ascertain which members of the social network are the most important to the person (with respect to the pain problem), and evaluate how their responses and actions influence the person.

Q1: Do you feel supported by other people?
Q2: Are you supported at home, in the workplace?

Useful Management Strategies: Address beliefs; Engage the significant other as rehabilitation 'collaborator'.

Perception of stressful job demands refers to the person's belief that their job is 'stressful'. This means that they believe it demands more from them than they are willing or capable to give.

Evaluation: Identify the person's perception of stressful elements in their job, and evaluate how realistic this is.

Q1: Are there stressful elements to your job that you find difficult?
Q2: What might help you cope better during an average day at work?

Useful Management Strategies: Cognitive therapy approach to address perception; or, negotiate job modifications.

Lack of job accommodations/modified work refers to the absence of opportunity to stay at work, or resume work, with the help of transitional work arrangements (work organisation or work tasks).

Workplace accommodations can provide the person with the opportunity to maintain, or regain, their regular work habits and relationships with supervisors and co-workers. They are usually temporary. There are two major types: (1) changes in work organisation such as using a different schedule for work, or for example allowing someone who cannot drive or use public transport to work at home during the transitional period, or exchange problematic secondary tasks for part of another employee's job description; and, (2) changes in the biomechanical aspects of the job such as modifying the physical environment, or changing the job tasks or workloads.

Evaluation: Identify what the person can do, with less emphasis on what they cannot do (except for safety-sensitive issues), and identify job tasks that can be done. Look for practical ways to begin the return to work process, and use a graded approach when appropriate.

Q1: What parts of your job can you still do?
Q2: What do you need to talk to you supervisor about in order to resume working?

Useful Management Strategies: Establish appropriate workplace policies and procedures; (professional) Case management; Case conferences; Effective communication between key players.

Lack of employer communication with employees refers to an inadequate management style. Duration of time off work is reduced by contact between healthcare and the workplace, and between employer and absent workers.

Lack of effective communication is a major obstacle to vocational rehabilitation and the return to work process. In general it needs to be improved through the development and use of practical and effective methods.

Evaluation: Identify what communication has occurred, and between which key players.

Q1: Has your employer made contact with you since you stopped work?
Q2: Has there been any communication between healthcare providers and the workplace?

Useful Management Strategies: Stay in touch; Facilitate effective communication between key players; Use a written confidentiality waiver; (professional) Case management.

Misunderstandings and disagreements between key players refers to disagreements, or differences in approaches. This may occur, for example between an employee and the employer, or with a healthcare provider.

Disputes and disagreements can arise when communication between key players is lacking or ineffective, especially when they misunderstand each other.

Evaluation: Identify contradictory or conflicting approaches, and how these have come about.

Q1: Do you understand what has been planned to help you?
Q2: Does everyone know what the plan is?

Useful Management Strategies: Keep key players informed; Mediation.

Financial and compensation problems refers to a range of incentives and disincentives that might occur due to the provision of financial support to the person.

Evaluation: Identify financial disincentives to resuming work; delays in accessing income support or disputes over eligibility; history of claims for injuries or other pain problems; or, history of extended time off work due to previous injury or pain problem.

Q1: Do you feel encouraged or discouraged to return to activity/work?
Q2: What (if anything) is holding you back?

Useful Management Strategies: Provide clear and accurate information; (professional) Case management.

Process delays refer to a range of potential problems that result in the person experiencing delay. This might be due to administrative mistakes, waiting lists for healthcare or other appointments, delays in claim acceptance or accessing income support, or disputes over eligibility of a claim.

Evaluation: Identify any delays, and associated distress and frustration.

Q1: Are you waiting for anything to be done to help you?
Q2: What is it?

Useful Management Strategies: (professional) Case management.

Overreactions to sensationalist media reports refers to information in the public domain heralding the possibility of new treatments with an over-hyped description of their effectiveness and suggestion of impending availability.

Expectations that modern medicine can cure or fix injuries and diseases commonly extend to musculoskeletal problems. This prevailing view is fuelled by a number of sources including enthusiastic clinicians and popular media reports. It can be intensified by news of new technological developments. The effect of expecting a biomedical cure can be to reinforce the notion that something is damaged, to encourage the belief that a cure exists, to strengthen the idea that pain must be completely relieved before commencing rehabilitation, and that a clinician is responsible for getting the person better.

Evaluation: Identify expectations of a 'quick fix' or 'miracle cure', and be alert for requests for new technologies

Q1: What do you think will help you recover?
Q2: Have you heard of any new treatments that are available?

Useful Management Strategies: Education and information; Encourage obtaining information from reliable sources; Address healthcare myths.

Unhelpful return to work policies or procedures refers to anything used by companies and workplaces that hinders the process.

Effective vocational rehabilitation requires healthcare that includes a specific focus on return to work and workplaces that are accommodating. In addition, there needs to be suitable communication, and coordination of the return to work process. Previous negative experience of workplace management, and absence of interest by an employer, or previous experience of ineffective case management, may contribute to negative expectations and beliefs.

Evaluation: Identify inadequate or lack of return to work 'culture' or policies that interfere with the actual process being used.

Q1: Is there a policy for helping someone return to work?
Q2: What does it involve?

Useful Management Strategies: Promote a 'Stay at Work' culture; Be committed to using the workplace as the site/vehicle for effective rehabilitation; Adopt a health promotion role to help dispel myths; Encourage workers to use self-help approaches, by allowing them to maintain activity as far as possible. Liaise with healthcare. Stay in touch with absentees. Avoid the '100% or nothing' rule.

USEFUL QUESTIONS for all key players to ask the person
- What do you think has caused your problem?
- What do you expect is going to happen?
- How are you coping with things?
- Is it getting you down?
- When do you think you'll get back to work?
- What can be done at work to help?

Effective interventions

All players
Information, advice, and reassurance
Promoting activity and work
Dispel myths (about pain, activity, and work)

Workplace
Transitional work arrangements - workload, schedule, tasks
Graded RTW programme
Negotiated job modifications
Case management

Healthcare
Address unhelpful thoughts
Relaxation training
Stress management training
Activity scheduling, progressive goals
Positive self-statements
Coping skills training
Problem-solving skills
Use relevant other as rehabilitation 'coach'
Desensitise fear of movement

making a difference

> **Communication is key** - Chang's story shows that identifying and tackling the Flags does make a difference, but all the players (including Chang) must act together.

Chang's story

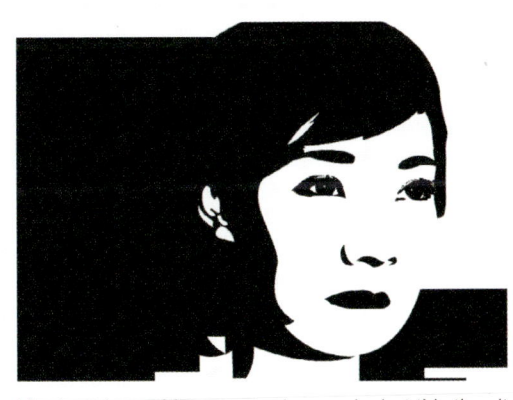

My shoulder problem cropped up again, but this time it seemed worse, so I asked the doc to check it out. Probably muscular he said, and it should settle OK - no need to stop doing anything. That made sense – my dad had an elbow problem, but it never laid him up. Anyway, after a week the shoulder wasn't any better and I couldn't manage at work. So back to the doc. He said I needed some rehab. So, I worked out a plan of action with my boss: agree a timeline > get some therapy > organise some help at work. One of my friends reckoned it must have been caused at work. That just had to be rubbish – I know I've got a physical job but I've been doing it for years and nothing's changed. I just needed some help to get my shoulder working again. The therapist agreed, and when I told her that my job could be made easier for a while, she said going back could actually help. The doc wrote to my boss about what I could manage, and when I went in to see the people at work they were really helpful. A few weeks later I was back at my usual work!

Helping people stay at/return to work depends on a combination of work-focused healthcare and an accommodating workplace. Both need to be coordinated. The imperative is to prevent development of negative psychosocial influences since these reduce the person's ability and willingness to participate in productive activity. Respond promptly when there is a lack of progress.

It is all too easy to overlook psychosocial factors during the very early stages of musculoskeletal problems. Even when they are noted, there is a tendency for little or nothing to be done about them.

To make a difference, some simple and straightforward things need to happen

- Routine and timely identification of the psychosocial obstacles
- Combining available information about the person, their workplace, and the context in order to formulate a practical Plan of Action
- Ensuring someone is responsible to make the Plan of Action happen
  - this could be healthcare provider, employer, case manager
    - but must be in conjunction with the person
    - communication + coordination ➜ plan

Developing a Plan of Action

Evaluation of a person reveals Flags. It is this knowledge that is used to develop a Plan to map out the basis for Action. The Plan is often simple: agreeing to a few straightforward goals and timelines lets the multiple players know who is doing what, and when – this enables them coordinate their actions.

> ### Chang's Plan of Action
>
> **My goals:** get back to modified duties in a couple of weeks, and usual work by the middle of next month.
>
> **What can I still do?** Most light physical stuff below shoulder height, provided I can rest occasionally.
>
> **Obstacles to return to work:** Difficulty keeping arms up or lifting heavy things, Uncertain about going back.
>
> **Who needs to do what, when?** This week – get doc's agreement to timeline; start treatment; sort out exercises to build up strength; go into work and discuss with supervisor how tasks can be eased. Next week – start on modified duties (part time for first few days); continue treatment/exercises. At 3 weeks – ramp up duties; keep supervisor informed on progress. At 4 weeks – move to full duties; keep supervisor informed.

'Making a difference depends on a combination of work-focused healthcare and an accommodating workplace'

action

what to do when - moving the Plan to Action

The Action requires:
- Appropriate healthcare intervention to deal with biomedical issues
- Healthcare that supports, and does not hinder, early return to activity/work
- Communication between the players to make it happen on time
- Workplace facilitation to ease the worker back to usual duties

But – these elements must be delivered simultaneously – they must be interwoven – they cannot be sequential.

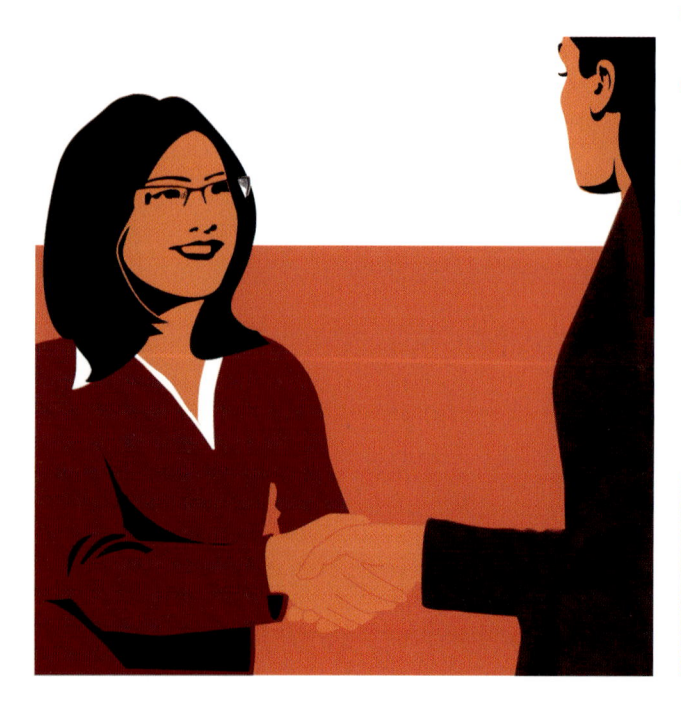

General principles:
- The intervention must address the identified Flags and obstacles, using both healthcare and workplace interventions.
- Interventions can address psychosocial factors, such as beliefs, fears, and avoidance behaviours.
- Psychosocial interventions such as problem-solving training and coping strategies can usefully supplement exercises and information/advice, and contribute to increasing activity.
- An accommodating workplace can be the key to work retention and early return to work.

Specific principles:
- Involve the workplace setting if possible, rather than the clinic alone.
- Ensure (through communication) that all players know what Actions are to be done, by whom, and when.

Evaluating progress:
- Audit goals using objective measures
  - record observed behaviours (e.g. hours at work, duration of sitting tolerance, return to usual job etc)
  - avoid subjective approaches, such as 'how are you feeling?' - ask instead 'what have you been doing?'

Interventions to address psychosocial factors are more effective, and use fewer resources when they are delivered early.

Psychologists are usually not needed. These principles can be adopted and used by all key players.

Workplace and healthcare goals: they may change with time.

Workplace

Enabling early return to work may require alterations to the way the job is done. These transitional work arrangements can involve both physical and organizational aspects. The important thing is that they are a temporary facilitator. They need to be reviewed on a regular basis and removed at the earliest opportunity.

Any worker who stops work due to a musculoskeletal problem should return to the same job with the same employer (SJSE): this is usually a realistic goal. On the relatively rare occasions when this fails, or is an inappropriate occupational goal, the appropriate target goal can be selected from the following hierarchy: Modified job, same employer (SJSE-Modified); Different job, same employer (DJSE); Same job, different employer (SJDE); Modified job, different employer (SJDE-Modified); Different job, different employer (DJDE); Vocational and/or academic retraining.

Healthcare

Immediately following onset of a musculoskeletal problem, the goal is to remain as active as possible, with early return to work. When recovery is slow, the goal is to obtain the maximal level of function and the person is expected to participate actively in managing their problem. Should the problem become persistent the goal may change to achieving the optimal level of participation.

Individual

The role of the individual invariably changes over time, and should move explicitly from being a passive recipient of healthcare and assistance, to active participation. It is important to ensure that significant others (e.g. spouse, family member) understand the problem and share the same goals, beliefs and commitment to the plan of action.

Communication

Clear communication among the players is essential in devising a plan: without adequate communication, effective action is impossible. But, many organisational and statutory systems actually get in the way - Black Flags are rife. Seen simply, the workplace must communicate with the worker and healthcare must communicate with the workplace (both are needed to facilitate work retention and return to work). To overcome obstacles it is essential to share information: a simple effective tool is the confidentiality waiver – the worker gives explicit written permission for (selected) people at the workplace to talk freely with the health professional(s) in order to figure out when and how the workplace can best accommodate the worker.

Workplace accommodations

Often people return to their usual job without any need for modifications. Maybe because they have fully recovered, or the job does not place demands on the particular muscles and joints concerned. However, for the worker with work-relevant symptoms, reasonable accommodation is imperative. Modified work should only be offered when required. The modifications should be devised with the worker's help and agreement, using a problem-solving approach.

In most cases modified work should be a temporary arrangement, and usually for a short period – they are a transitional arrangement simply to enable early return to a job that would otherwise be challenging while the person recovers. An offer of modified work does not imply that the original job carried significant risks or was (necessarily) the cause of the problem. Assuming suitable risk controls are in place, modified work is not an indictment of the original job for a fit, healthy worker – if there are any concerns, a re-assessment is in order.

The required modifications will depend on the balance between the work demands, the health problem and the person. Consider both the physical demands of the work and the way it is organized: the basic idea is to reduce exposure to tasks that the worker cannot comfortably do because of the musculoskeletal problem.

Some examples of helpful workplace accommodations to tackle common obstacles:

- Alter the work tasks or physical environment to reduce physical demands – e.g. reduce reaching; provide seating; reduce weights; reduce pace of work/frequency; enable help from co-workers; job enlargement (added task variety).

- Alter the work organisation – e.g. flexible start/finish times; reduced work hours/days; additional rest breaks; graded return to work (starting at achievable level, and increase on a regular quota, or start with a short week).

- Change the job – e.g. allow someone who cannot drive or use public transport to work at home during the transitional period, or exchange problematic secondary tasks for part of another employee's job description.

- Flexibility – e.g. schedule daily planning sessions with a co-worker at the start of each day to develop achievable goals; allow reasonable time to attend healthcare appointments.

Taking action – Kamala's story shows how the supervisor can make things happen

Kamala's role

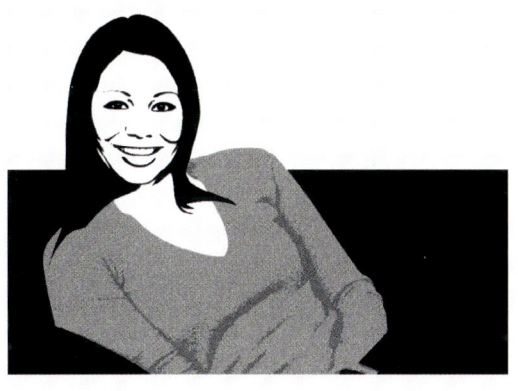

We're a small company without formal occ health cover. The senior management have taken advice and introduced a simple protocol for managing musculoskeletal problems. It's my job to put it into action. Basically, I coordinate the return to work process – I act as a case manager with support from professionals. I get informed at day one of absence, and stay in contact. I liaise with the doctor, and also send our people to a local clinic – they're well versed in occ health matters. They do an assessment and tell me what my colleague can do (we use a confidentiality waiver). They help me figure out how best to help my colleague back to work. They point out the obstacles and what needs to be done to overcome them, as well as giving treatment. I devise the Plan with my colleague and we sort out any work modifications as a team. I use information leaflets to help explain things and bust the myths. It works well!

'Communication and workplace facilitation are key to success'

timing
shifting the recovery curve

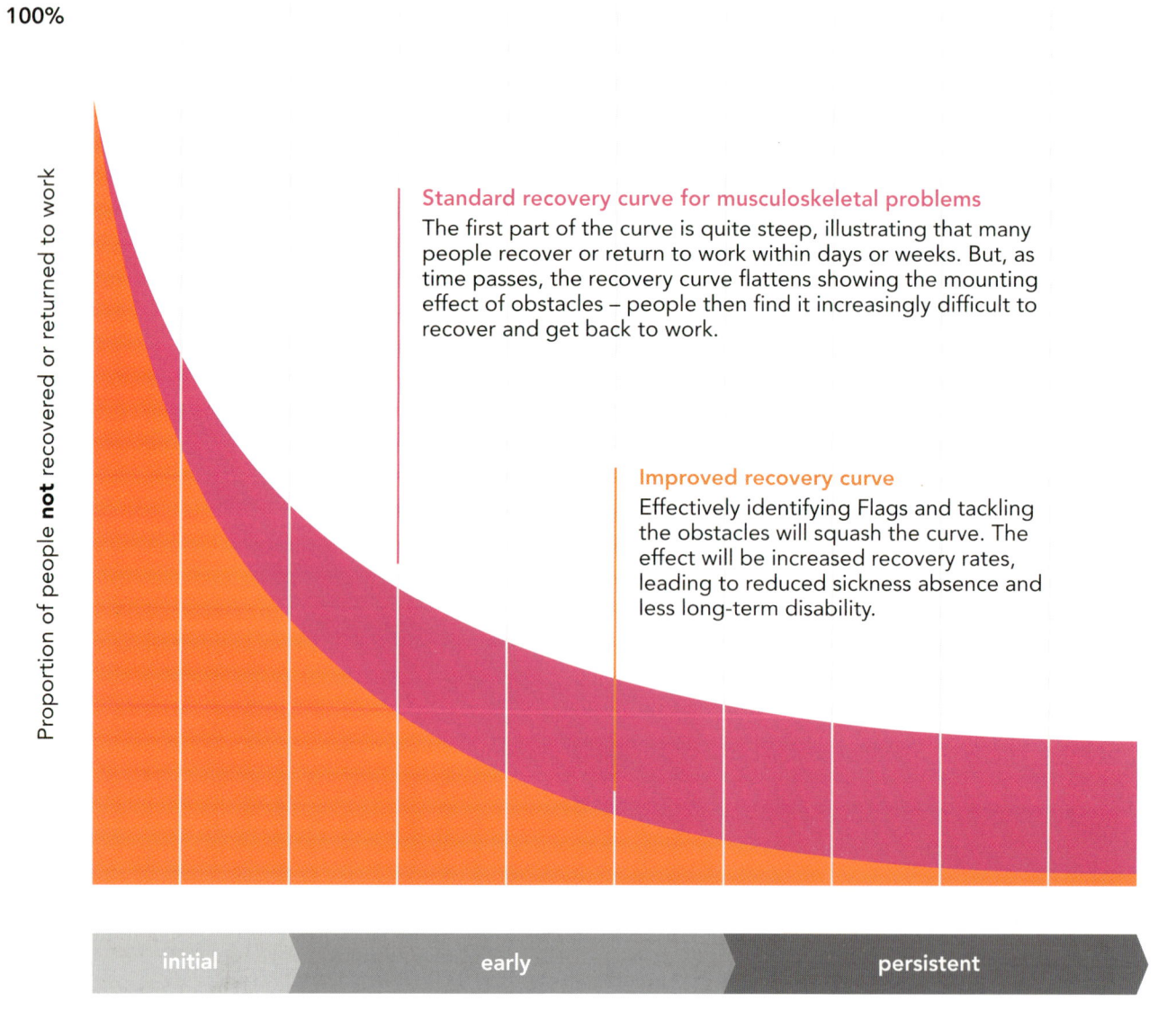

100%

Proportion of people **not** recovered or returned to work

Standard recovery curve for musculoskeletal problems
The first part of the curve is quite steep, illustrating that many people recover or return to work within days or weeks. But, as time passes, the recovery curve flattens showing the mounting effect of obstacles – people then find it increasingly difficult to recover and get back to work.

Improved recovery curve
Effectively identifying Flags and tackling the obstacles will squash the curve. The effect will be increased recovery rates, leading to reduced sickness absence and less long-term disability.

initial → early → persistent

Timeline - increasing time since onset of symptoms (or going off work)

Implications for Evaluation
Difficulties increase over time. Usually the impact of psychosocial factors increases, and new issues begin to emerge.

This is important both for sequential evaluation, and the allocation of intervention resources.

A stepped approach to both evaluation and intervention is required.

Initial phase, within about first 2 weeks (often referred to as 'acute')
- Focus – symptomatic relief, maintain activity level.
- Resources - high proportion returns to activity and work in initial period: intensive resources not required.

Early phase, between about 2 and 12 weeks ('sub-acute')
- Focus – early return to work/activity: healthcare and workplace management needs a consistent work focus: workplace must be accommodating.
- Resources - step up input and resources: this is the optimal time to prevent the development of long-term consequences, including work loss.

Persistent phase, after about 12 weeks ('chronic')
- Focus – achieving maximal level of function and participation: consider shifting goals.
- Resources – requires more resources, and goals more difficult to achieve.

stepped care
just what's needed when its needed

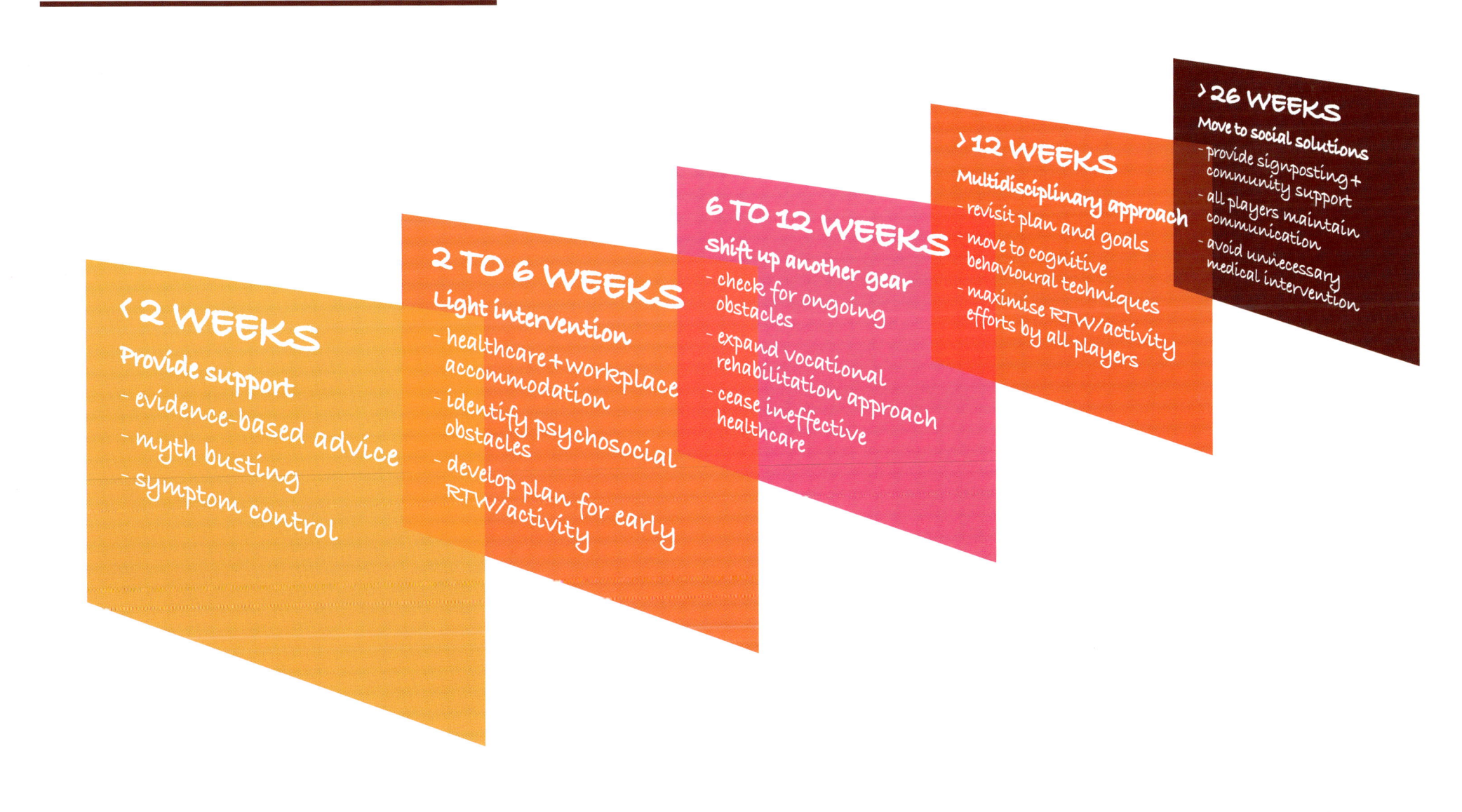

< 2 WEEKS
Provide support
- evidence-based advice
- myth busting
- symptom control

2 TO 6 WEEKS
Light intervention
- healthcare + workplace accommodation
- identify psychosocial obstacles
- develop plan for early RTW/activity

6 TO 12 WEEKS
Shift up another gear
- check for ongoing obstacles
- expand vocational rehabilitation approach
- cease ineffective healthcare

> 12 WEEKS
Multidisciplinary approach
- revisit plan and goals
- move to cognitive behavioural techniques
- maximise RTW/activity efforts by all players

> 26 WEEKS
Move to social solutions
- provide signposting + community support
- all players maintain communication
- avoid unnecessary medical intervention

initial → early → persistent

Timeframes - progressively fewer people remain as time passes - step times are approximate

© Kendall & Burton 2009 Full guide: www.tsoshop.co.uk/flags

stepped care approach - *timelines & actions for the key players*

	At All Times	Symptoms Reported	Healthcare Sought	Off Work	Return To Work
EMPLOYER (management and supervisors) > accommodate the worker, facilitate return to work, and have policies to ensure communication with healthcare professionals <flexibility>	**All players can, at all times:** > Promote a Stay at Work culture. > Be committed to using the workplace as the site for effective rehabilitation. > Adopt a health promotion role to dispel myths. > Encourage workers to use self-help approaches, by allowing them to maintain activity. > Ensure risk assessments are up to date and controls in place.	Ensure line manager or supervisor talks to the person about workload, tasks, and/or schedule. Note presence of significant Blue Flags. Identify any organisational obstacles to recovery. Provide evidence-based information and advice. Consider the work, workplace, and healthcare needs of the person to help them stay in work. Identify suitable tasks and work hours if required. Obtain medical advice in face of severe or persistent symptoms.	Note presence of significant Blue Flags. Provide advice as per evidence-based guidance. Assign someone to maintain contact with the person. Maintain Stay at Work approach. Offer modified work. Use written confidentiality waiver.	Educate and inform staff about effective return to work (RTW)* approaches. Assign responsibility to ensure RTW is discussed early, and implemented practically. Agree a RTW plan. Obtain reliable (e.g. occupational health) advice if needed. Maintain regular contact. Encourage attendance at work meetings and social events. Discuss transitional work arrangements: update risk assessment if appropriate.	Implement graded RTW plan. Obtain reliable (e.g. occupational health) advice needed. Monitor RTW progress.
HEALTHCARE PROVIDER (family physician, therapists, occupational health) > provide work-focused care, offer positive advice about work and health, and liaise with employer <communication>		Open lines of communication. Facilitate communication between key players. Use written confidentiality waiver.	Note presence of significant Yellow Flags. Provide advice as per evidence-based guidelines. Encourage Stay at Work. Reassure and explain typical pattern of discomfort. Advise the person and employer on work tasks and hours, activities, and symptom relief. Assist people to understand what healthcare can and cannot provide (i.e. healthcare is often not the full answer). Downplay work attribution. Provide evidence-based diagnosis, including consideration of Red Flags.	Encourage activity and participation. Agree a RTW plan. Provide a 'fit note', emphasise ability not disability.	Review progress objectively. Encourage activity and participation.
CASE MANAGER or EMPLOYMENT ADVISOR > support and advise the other players and facilitate cooperation to overcome obstacles <coordination>			Note presence of significant Black Flags. Provide evidence-based information and advice. Encourage Stay at Work. Objectively monitor outcomes of healthcare provided.	Develop RTW plan negotiated with all the other players. Ensure timely and appropriate healthcare provided. Liaise directly with healthcare providers and employer. Ask doctor to provide a 'fit note' that emphasises ability not disability.	Ensure timely start for RTW. Set RTW expectations with the person and employer. Liaise with healthcare provider and employer regarding RTW plan. Monitor RTW progress. Adjust RTW approach if required. Be cost-aware and ensure resources used efficiently.

»» timeline »»

'The longer the duration of symptoms/absence, the more intense the intervention'

	2-4 WEEKS	6-8 WEEKS	about 12 WEEKS	about 26 WEEKS
EMPLOYER should	Evaluate Blue Flags/obstacles. Maintain contact with absentee – tag to ensure followed-up. Formulated individualised, targeted management strategy: Plan of Action. Liaise with healthcare provider to offer workplace modifications and get RTW prediction – request a 'fit note'.	Re-evaluate Blue Flags /obstacles. Intensify efforts to facilitate RTW. Suggest all parties meet to discuss employment options. Provide temporary modified work tasks/ organisation - review regularly. Liaise with healthcare. Consider specialist occupational health input.	Review progress, and re-evaluate Blue Flags/obstacles. Consider refining Plan of Action. Review modified work, adjustments to tasks or work organisation. Consider temporary re-deployment, or need for re-training. Get specialist occupational health input.	Offer re-deployment or goal oriented job training. Review worker's status with specialist occupational health provider. Reiterate worker's worth to company. Emphasise commitment to liaising with other players to facilitate RTW.
HEALTHCARE PROVIDER should	Evaluate Yellow Flags. Select cases for psychosocial management (without interfering with clinical treatments). Formulate individualised, targeted management strategy. Encourage self-help approach. Liaise with workplace to develop RTW plan. Suggest suitable job modifications. Issue 'fit note' when appropriate.	Re-evaluate Yellow Flags and identify ongoing obstacles to participation and RTW. Intensify efforts to restore activity and RTW: positive encouragement. Incorporate cognitive behavioural principles. Cease ineffective therapies (to prevent passivity, dependence). Liaise with workplace: give 'fit note'. Support and encourage work.	Evaluate progress, and re-evaluate Yellow Flags and obstacles. Consider refining and/or modifying goals and targets. Encourage the person to adopt self-management approach. Support and encourage work. Advise on ability to work.	Emphasise independence, self-efficacy (sense of mastery), best sustainable level of function, and highest quality of life. Establish sustainable level of ongoing healthcare and avoid unnecessary investigations or invasive procedures. Maintain communication with workplace.
CASE MANAGER or EMPLOYMENT ADVISOR should	Evaluate Black Flags/obstacles. Liaise directly with healthcare provider and workplace. Check Yellow and Blue Flags are being evaluated. Ensure maximum RTW effort by all key players: facilitate communication. Manage expectations. Make cost-effective decisions and manage resources.	Re-evaluate Black and Blue Flags/ obstacles. Cease ineffective therapies (to prevent passivity, dependence). Ensure maximum RTW effort by all key players. Consider a 'light' multidisciplinary programme that delivers pain management and vocational rehabilitation using cognitive behavioural principles.	Evaluate progress, and re-evaluate Black Flags/obstacles. Provide support and encouragement to maintain and improve work capacity. Ensure maximum RTW effort by all key players. Move to a full multidisciplinary programme that delivers cognitive-behavioural pain management and vocational rehabilitation.	Reassess ongoing healthcare needs and redirect as necessary. Identify transferable skills. Provide signposting to job-seeking support and guidance.

»» timeline »»

© Kendall & Burton 2009 Full guide: www.tsoshop.co.uk/flags

advice for workers with muscle and joint problems
helping you to stay active and working

1. important information
- Activity and work are good for physical and mental health
- Muscle and joint problems are very common – pretty much everyone has them at some stage during their life
- These problems can be distressing and may make life difficult for a while
- Serious disease or injury with lasting damage is very rare
- Most episodes settle quickly, but the symptoms may crop up again
- It's best to stay active and continue working, or get back soon

2. identify obstacles to your recovery
Various things can get in the way of recovery and getting back to work and activity

Personal obstacles involve how you feel and think:-
Unhelpful attitudes and beliefs about health and work • Uncertainty • Anxiety and depression • Loss of routine and work habits

Work-related obstacles can block your return to work:-
Loss of contact with work • Negative attitudes by people at work • Lack of job accommodations or modified work • Misunderstandings and disagreements between you, your employer, and doctor/therapist)

Health-related obstacles can confuse and delay:-
Conflicting advice • waiting lists • prolonged sick leave • ineffective treatments

things to watch out for
You are unlikely to recover and return to work if you
→ Believe there is something seriously wrong
→ Are unable to accept reassurance and help
→ Avoid activity in case it makes things worse
→ Get withdrawn and depressed
→ Are fearful and uncertain about going back to work

The longer you are off work or not doing your usual activities, the harder it is to get back

3. make a plan to be active and working
The key is communication and action. There are two main issues:

Recovery depends on working with the health professionals who are helping you, and on your own motivation and effort. Treatment can help to reduce your symptoms, but you are the one who has to get active – see activity as part of your treatment

Ask yourself: What can I do to be a 'coper' and not an 'avoider'?

Returning to work depends on you and your employer working together, and that needs communication. The key thing is to stay in touch with the people at work – figure out what's needed to help you return

Ask yourself: What obstacles are getting in the way of my going back to work, and who do I need to talk to about overcoming these (through problem-solving and negotiation)

4. action!
Putting your plan into action:

Take control - Take responsibility for your recovery, making best use of available help

Set realistic goals - Give yourself a clear timeline for getting back to work and activity. Use weeks, not months

List what you can do - Have a 'can-do' approach, and avoid dwelling on what you can't do easily at present. You'll find you can do a lot of things – at work and leisure

Talk with your health professional – Discuss what you can do: work out ways to get active and back to work. Give them permission to talk with your employer

Increase activity – Do a little more each day for a little longer. Pace yourself: do no more on good days and no less on bad days

Changing your attitude and improving motivation – Don't get gloomy or anxious. Getting active will improve your confidence and you'll feel more positive

Talk with your employer – If your employer has not been in touch, make the first move. Temporary changes to your job are one of the best ways of making it possible to get back to work: sort out what's needed with your line manager

Put it all together – Make sure that you and your doctor and your employer all know what is happening and what you are planning. Tell them you want help to be a *coper*

© Kendall & Burton 2009 Full guide: www.tsoshop.co.uk/flags